HERBS FOR RHEUMATISM AND ARTHRITIS

Describes twenty-five herbs for treating rheumatism and arthritis by ridding the body of excess acids and purifying the blood. With supplementary advice on dietetics, vitamins, Epsom salts baths and compresses, exercise and relaxation.

By the same author

HERBS TO SOOTHE YOUR NERVES
HERBS FOR CLEARING THE SKIN
HERBS FOR FEMININE AILMENTS
HERBS FOR PROSTATE AND BLADDER TROUBLES
HERBS FOR RHEUMATISM AND ARTHRITIS

HERBS FOR RHEUMATISM AND ARTHRITIS

by
SARAH BECKETT

Drawings by Jill Fry

THORSONS PUBLISHERS LIMITED
Wellingborough, Northamptonshire

First published 1975
Sixth Impression 1985

ISBN 0 7225 0300 8

Printed and bound in Great Britain by
Richard Clay (The Chaucer Press) Ltd.,
Bungay, Suffolk.

CONTENTS

1.

ABOUT RHEUMATISM AND ARTHRITIS

A report by the Arthritis and Rheumatism Council states that about 5½ million people in this country suffering from rheumatic complaints consult their doctors every year. This is more than a tenth of the population.

People from all walks of life succumb to arthritis and rheumatism and the aim of this book is to introduce natural herbal medicines as a means of relief, and in many cases, cure.

Many years ago all aches and pains were put under the heading of rheumatism. As time went on and more research was done, it was found necessary and helpful, to break down this disease into two main divisions, the aches and pains of the muscles, and those of the joints.

Hence we now have:

1. Muscular rheumatism, which includes fibrositis, etc.
2. Rheumatism in the joints, which is known as arthritis, and includes osteo-arthritis, rheumatoid arthritis and gout.

Muscular rheumatism is perhaps the most common. The pains vary and may be sharp or dull and aching. They occur most frequently in the back, neck and shoulders, and often nodules can be felt when treatment is being given.

Tensions and strains can bring these pains to life because when the patient is tense, so are his muscles, and it is then that they make themselves felt.

Driving a car for long periods will cause tensions across the shoulders and back of the neck, and pain will develop. Typing will often do the same thing. Many household jobs in the kitchen will create trouble; ironing, for instance, will cause the right shoulder to become painful if the ironing board is not at the right height; cooking on a surface that is either too high or too low will strain and tense the neck and shoulder muscles, and so on.

Arthritis is rheumatism of the joints. Osteo-arthritis is due, in the main, to wear and tear of the joints. By this is meant that because joints move, the bone surfaces which form the joints, rub on each other, and it is inevitable that if they are used too much they wear, one on the other. This applies to people who do jobs involving excessive repetitive action using the same joint, or joints. After a certain amount of wear and tear the joint is not so efficient, and an inflammatory condition may flare up, causing pain and swelling.

Almost everybody over the age of fifty has this wear and tear, but often it causes little or no inconvenience. The gristle lining the joints becomes thin, and the bones round the edge grow knobby, and the knobs may get in the way. It is easy to understand that overweight can worsen some conditions, especially when the trouble is in the hips and knees.

Rheumatoid arthritis is swelling and inflammation of the tissue lining the joints; as this heals tough fibres form, making movement difficult and pulling the joints out of line.

The intake of too much refined food, and too many foods which cause an acid reaction in the system is also one of the chief factors and this is dealt with under *Supplementary Advice* at the end of the book.

Gout is due to excessive uric acid in the system which may be deposited in the joints, and inflammation sets in with excruciating pain. It is common in the big toe joint and cries of 'Mind my foot' are common from patients thus affected. But it must be emphasized that gout can and does affect many other joints.

There is usually an inherited tendency in rheumatic troubles, and this can sometimes be traced back through several generations. The diseases themselves are not inherited, but the soil or bloodstream in which rheumatism and arthritis can thrive, may be handed down from one generation to another, unless it is changed by natural remedies that can attack the cause.

The two most common factors that trigger off these painful ailments are:

1. The stress and strain of modern living.
2. The daily intake of foods that are toxic and very acid in character. Both will be dealt with later in the book.

2.

WHY HERBS CAN HELP

It is difficult to know why many more patients do not take advantage of herbal medicine and why more doctors do not examine this form of treatment.

Herbs are as old as mankind. Indeed it is said, 'herbs are for the healing of the nations' and it is interesting to note that those indigenous to the country are often able to clear up the sicknesses peculiar to that particular climate and environment.

The healing plants are safe and produce no side-effects. They are gentle and may be given to all ages and for all conditions. They are foods as well as medicines as they contain starches, sugars and protein. In addition they supply mineral salts in the minute quantities that the body can absorb, plus natural vitamins and other elements vital to health and these are all in their natural form.

Another interesting point about herbal medicines is that each plays more than one role. For instance, Prickly Ash is a stimulant, alterative, tonic and diaphoretic, which means that it produces energy, helps to renew tissues, gives tone to the body — thus producing a feeling of well-being, and produces perspiration.

Because herbs have such a wide range of action, they are strongly recommended in the treatment of rheumatic and arthritic conditions. They may help to rid the body of excess acids, which goes a long way towards clearing up these aches and pains; many herbs are excellent blood purifiers, despatching the impure waste products through the urine, bowels or skin; and there are those that soothe the aches and pains of muscles and bones.

How much wiser it is to take medicine from the plants of the meadows and hillside, 'weeds' most people call them, containing natural ingredients, rather than drugs which, generally, mask the condition by deadening pain and palliating sickness; in addition they often create side-effects which can put extra strain on vital organs of the body.

We can be certain that in the days to come, more and more people will turn to herbal medicine, homoeopathy and acupuncture because there is so much dissatisfaction with drug therapy.

Herbs cleanse the whole system. They are gentle. They are safe. They are natural.

3.

AGRIMONY
(Agrimonia Eupatoria)

Also known as Cocklebur and Stickwort.

Description: This is a common plant growing abundantly in the borders of fields, by ditches and hedges and in woods. The leaves are long, dented at the edges, green above, greenish and hairy underneath; the plant grows to from two to three feet high, with smaller leaves at the top. The small yellow flowers grow one above the other in long yellow spikes. They bloom in July and August. The fruit is small, pointed at the base and broadening towards the top, ribbed, with hooked bristles at the apex. Each fruit contains two seeds. The taste is astringent and slightly bitter.

Part used: The herb.

It bears the titles Cocklebur and Sticklewort because the seedpods cling, by the hooked end of the stiff hairs, to the clothing of people and to the coats of animals.

Fernie says that Agrimony tea is drunk as a beverage at table in France.

In the time of Chaucer, when we find the name appearing as Egrimoyne, it was used with Mugwort and vinegar for 'a bad back'.

Culpeper says, 'It is a most admirable remedy for such whose lives are annoyed either by heat or cold. The liver is the former of blood and blood the nourisher of the body, and agrimony a strengthener of the liver.'

This is a most helpful remedy in all arthritic and rheumatic conditions if taken regularly over a long period.

Directions for use: One pint of boiling water

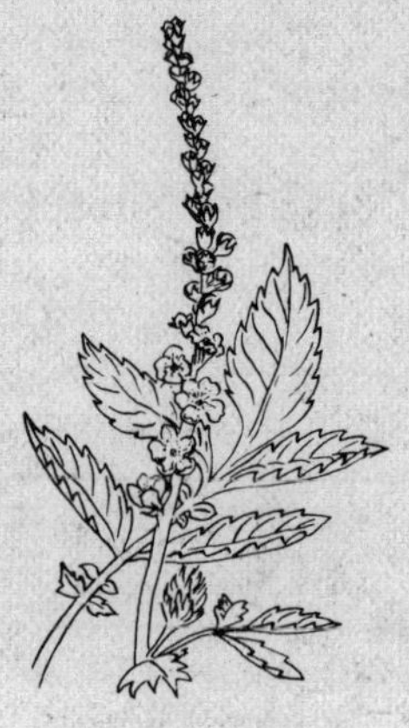

Agrimony

should be poured on to 1 oz of the herb and when it is cold and strained, take a wineglassful three times daily.

4.

ANGELICA
(Angelica Archangelica)

Also known as Garden Angelica and Master-wort.

Description: It is common in gardens in England and it also grows wild. The plant grows to about 6 feet tall on large hollow stems, the bottom leaves are large, broad and pointed with serrated edges, on short stalks. The upper leaves are similar but smaller. There are large heads made up of tiny greenish-white flowers. The root is from 2-4 inches long and 1 to 2 inches thick; when cut the fresh root yields a thick yellow juice. The smell is fragrant, the taste aromatic.

Part used: Root, seeds and herbs, but mostly an infusion from the herb.

Angelica has been known for many centuries and its virtues are praised by writers of old for curing every conceivable malady.

Mrs Grieve says: 'In Courland, Livonia and the low lakelands of Pomerania and East Prussia, wild growing Angelica abounds; there, in early summer-time, it has been the custom among the peasants to march into the towns carrying Angelica flower stems and to offer them for sale chanting some ancient ditty in Lettish words, so antiquated as to be unintelligible even to the singers themselves. The chanted words and the tune are learnt in childhood, and may be attributed to a survival of some Pagan Festival with which the plant was originally associated.'

Fernie says: 'Angelica came to this country from northern latitudes in 1568. The aromatic stems are grown abundantly near London in moist fields for the use of confectioners. These stems, when candied, are sold as a favourite sweetmeat.'

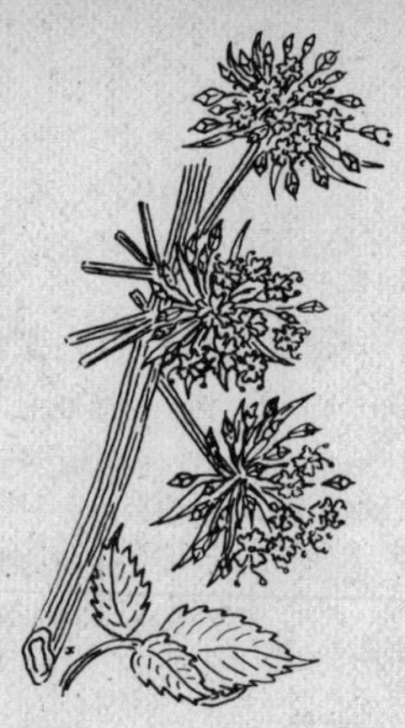

Angelica

Culpeper says: '. . . the distilled water applied to places pained with gout or sciatica doth give a great deal of ease.'

The stem and roots, if pulverized, yield a yellow juice, which becomes, when dried, a valuable medicine beneficial in chronic rheumatism and gout.

Directions for use: One pint of boiling water should be poured on to 1 oz of the powdered root, and when it is cold and strained, take a wineglassful three times daily. The same directions should be followed if using 1 oz of the dried herb instead of the powdered root; it should be taken in the same way.

5.

ASH
(Fraxinus excelsior)

Also known as Common Ash, European Ash, Weeping Ash.

Description: This is a tall, handsome tree, common in Britain and distinguished by the light grey bark and large compound ash-coloured leaves divided into four to eight pairs of lance-shaped leaflets topped by a single one.

Part used: The bark and leaves.

The timber of this tree is most valuable. It grows very quickly but the toughness and elasticity of the wood is said to surpass every tree in Europe.

In olden days it was used for spears and bows and today the wood is used extensively. The wood of the Ash tree is so elastic that a joist of it will bear more before it breaks than one made from any other tree.

The leaves are most useful in cases of arthritis

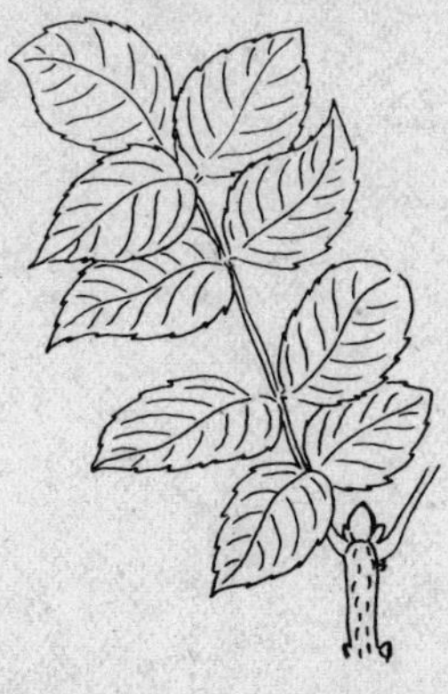

Ash

and rheumatism because of their laxative action. It is helpful when the joints are painful.

Directions for use: An infusion should be made by pouring 1 pint of boiling water on to 1 oz of the leaves and when it is cold and strained, take a wineglassful three times daily.

6.

BLACK COHOSH
(Cimicifuga racemosa)

Also known as Black Snakeroot, Bugbane, Rattleroot, Rattleweed, Squawroot.

Description: Black Cohosh grows in herbaceous borders so long as it has plenty of sunshine, but its home is America, Canada and Kashmir. It has snake-like cream flowers – and the root is thick, hard and knotty with short lateral branches.

Part used: The root.

One of the old herbalists, Dr W.A. Spurgeon of America, says of this herb: 'It is of special value in the treatment of muscular rheumatism, and for such it is being recommended. . . .'

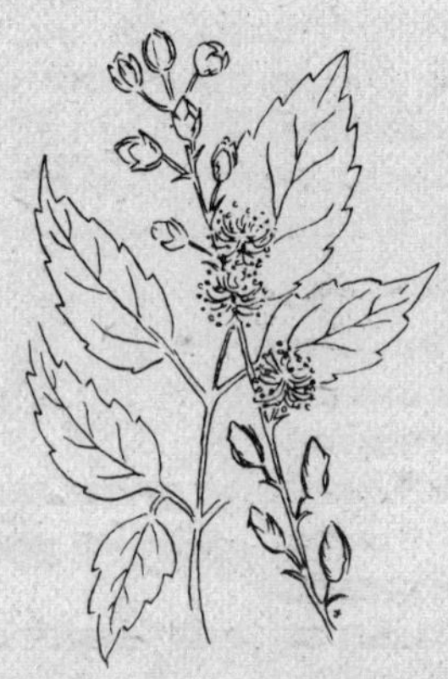

Black Cohosh

He also says: 'While Cimicifuga enjoys its greatest reputation as a remedy for chorea and muscular rheumatism, it is perhaps just as valuable for its action on the pelvic structures, and particularly uterine disturbances; it relieves the neuralgic and rheumatic pains in this region very promptly.'

This herb also acts on the central nervous system, the heart and the circulation.

Black Cohosh should be thought of when the pain is in the belly of the muscles. It is useful in intercostal rheumatism, rheumatic pains in muscles of back and neck, and aching in limbs with muscular soreness.

Directions for use: 10-15 drops of the liquid extract should be taken in a little water three times daily.

7.

BLADDERWRACK
(Fucus vesiculosus)

Also known as Kelpware, Our Lady's Wrack, Bladder Fucus and Cutweed.

Description: This is found on most of our sea coasts, in heavy brown masses of coarse-looking seaweed. It is fronded, flat, forked and blackish, about ½ inch broad and 1 or 2 feet long, with a midrib and oval bladders, usually in pairs.

Part used: The dried plant.

An analysis of Bladderwrack has shown it to contain an empyreumatic oil, sulphur, earthly salts, some iron and iodine.

Bladderwrack is a useful manure for potatoes and other crops and is gathered for this purpose all round the British coasts.

The fluid extract of this seaweed has a long

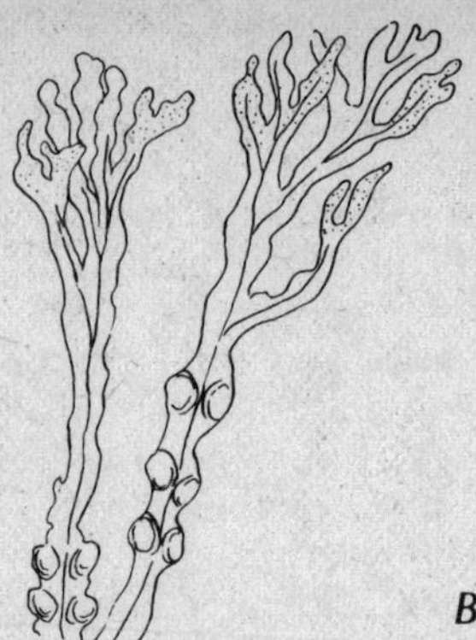

Bladderwrack

standing reputation of safely diminishing an excess of personal fat.

In 1862 Dr Duchesne-Duparc found while experimenting in cases of chronic psoriasis, that weight was reduced, without injuring health, and subsequently used Bladderwrack for this latter purpose.

Bladderwrack will relieve rheumatic pains and is especially useful in arthritic cases if the patient is overweight.

Directions for use: The fluid extract should be taken three times daily in doses of from 1-4 teaspoonsful.

8.

BUCKBEAN
(Menyanthes trifolata)

Also known as Bog-bean, Marsh Trefoil, Water Shamrock.

Description: It grows on marsh ground and on the margins of woodlands. The leaves grow alternately on stalks. There are three equal leaflets, inversely egg-shaped and wavelike. The flower stalk

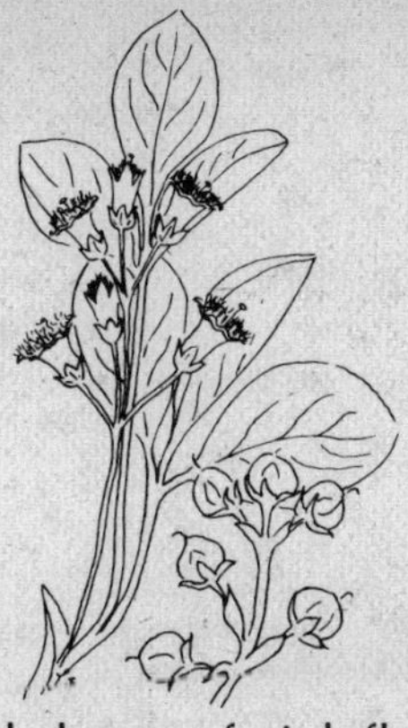

Buckbean

supports a stalked cluster of pink flowers, fringed within the corolla. It creeps in every direction as it has long rooting stems.

Part used: The herb.

The generic name Menyanthes is from two Greek words meaning 'month' and 'flower' It was the name given by Linnaeus and some think that the plant was so called because it remains in flower for a month. However, it often blooms during May, June and July!

The leaves of this herb have been substituted for hops in brewing beer.

It is also used as an herb tobacco.

Buckbean is a splendid tonic and most useful in the treatment of chronic rheumatism and lumbago.

An excellent combination for gout, rheumatism and lumbago is Buckbean, Yarrow, Pellitory-of-the-Wall and Cayenne pepper.

Directions for use: One oz of the dried, or 2 oz of the fresh herb should be boiled in $1\frac{1}{2}$ pints of water down to 1 pint, and when it is strained take a wineglassful three times daily.

The combination should be made up as follows:

1 oz Buckbean
1 oz Yarrow
½ teaspoonful Pellitory-of-the-Wall
½ oz Cayenne pepper

The herbs should be boiled in 3 pints of water down to 1 quart. This should be strained and the hot infusion poured over the Cayenne pepper. A wineglassful may be taken four or five times daily.

9.

BURDOCK
(Arctium lappa)

Also known as Lappa Hill, Beggars Burr, Thorny Burr, Clotbur, Hardock, Larebur, Turkey Burr, Personata and Happy Major. The burs of this dock are sometimes called cockle buttons, cuckle buttons, beggar's buttons.

Description: This plant grows in large quantities in fairly damp places, along roadsides and about old buildings on waste ground. The root is brownish-grey, and has a slightly sweet taste. The stem grows from 3-4 feet; the leaves are large, often 18-20

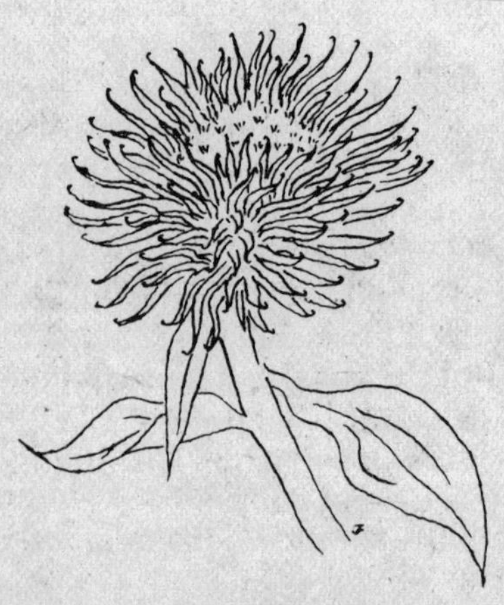

Burdock

inches long, and look rather like those of rhubarb; they are whitish underneath. The flowers are like thistles and purple in colour, they grow on short stems, often at the leaf joint. They are globular with burs that can stick to clothing. The fruits, (erroneously called seeds) are brownish-grey and wrinkled. The leaves and stems have a bitter taste.

Part used: The herb,root and seeds (fruits).

This plant gets its name of 'dock' from its large leaves; the 'bur' is supposed to be a contraction of the French *bourre*, from the Latin *burra*, a lock of wool, such as is often found entangled with it when sheep have passed by the growing plants.

The stalks, cut before the flower is open, and stripped of their rind, form a delicate vegetable, similar in flavour to Asparagus, and also make a tasty salad, eaten raw with oil and lemon juice.

Burdock has an old reputation for curing rheumatism, the large leaves being applied to the painful limb.

Sir Robert Walpole praised a decoction of the roots as a remedy for gout.

This herb is one of the best purifiers in herbal medicine, and therefore sufferers from any of the arthritic or rheumatic ailments must benefit from it.

Burdock is excellent for muscular rheumatism and arthritis in combination with Buckbean, Celery Seed, Meadowsweet and Yarrow.

Directions for use: Both root and seed may be taken as a decoction of 1 oz to 1½ pints of water boiled down to a pint. A wineglassful should be taken three or four times daily.

10-20 drops of the fluid extract may be taken in water three times daily.

A tea is made by infusing ½ oz of the herb in ¼ pint of boiling water for fifteen minutes; a wineglassful should be taken after every meal.

For the combination take:

½ oz Burdock
½ oz Buckbean
½ oz Celery seed
½ oz Meadowsweet
½ oz Yarrow

The herbs should be thoroughly mixed and simmered in 2½ pints of water for ten minutes. When cold and strained, a wineglassful should be taken three times daily.

10.

CELERY
(Apium graveolens)

Also known as Smallage, Marsh Parsley.

Description: This is cultivated in Britain. The wild variety grows in Southern Europe and has an unpleasant odour.

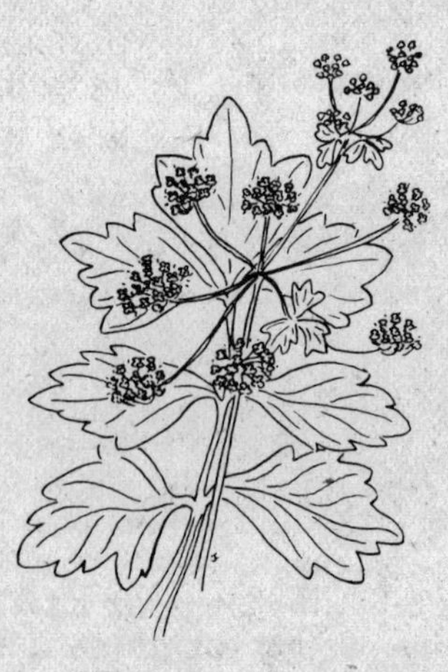

Celery

Part used: The seeds and stems.

The Romans adorned the heads of their guests, and the tombs of their dead with crowns of Smallage!

The Romanies cook celery in a little milk and then eat both. This, they claim, neutralizes uric acid, lactic acid and other acids in excess in the body, thus cleansing the muscular tissues.

Dr Fernie says: '. . . for relieving rheumatism wash the celery and cut it into small pieces and stew them well in a little water. Strain this and put aside . . . to be taken two or three tablespoonsful at a time. Dr Stacey Jones advises celery tea, hot and strong, with cream and sugar if desired, to be drunk by the cupful three or four times in the day, to abate neuralgia, and even sciatica, which it sometimes will do very speedily.'

Dr Pereira has shown that celery contains sulphur, which – Dr Fernie adds – is a known preventive of rheumatism.

Celery seeds may be sprinkled over vegetables and salads.

Celery is excellent for all sufferers from arthritis and rheumatism as it contains calcium, potassium, phosphorus, sodium and iron. It also contains vitamins A, B and C in addition to potash, sulphur, silicon, magnesium, apiol and an insulin ingredient. It has an alkaline reaction on the body.

Directions for use: It should be taken raw as often as possible and as described above.

The liquid extract may be obtained and from 5-10 drops taken three times daily.

11.

CENTAURY
(Erythraea centaurium)

Also known as Century, Centory, Feverwort.

Description: The stem is quadrangular, branched above, 8-12 inches high, with opposite oblong leaves with 3-5 longitudinal ribs. The flowers are pink with twisted anthers in pannicles. It grows on heaths and in dry pastures and also on cliffs by the sea. The taste is bitter.

Part used: The herb and leaves.

The genus was formerly called Chironia from the Centaur Chiron, who was famous in Greek mythology for his skill in medical herbs.

In a translation of an old mediaeval Latin poem by Macer, Centaury is mentioned (amongst other

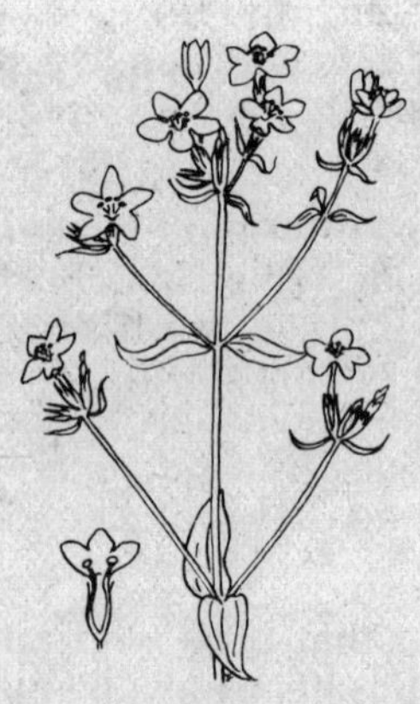

Centaury

herbs) as being powerful against 'wykked sperytis'.

Culpeper says: 'The herb is so safe you cannot fail in the using of it. Take it inwardly only for inward diseases, and apply it outwardly for outward complaints; it is very wholesome, but not very toothsome!'

He also says: '. . . and is very effective in all old pains of the joints, as the gout . . . '

This herb purifies the blood and is an excellent tonic. It should be thought of in muscular rheumatism.

Directions for use: 1 oz of the herb (and/or leaves) should be added to 1 pint of boiling water and when it is cool and strained take a wineglassful three times daily.

12.

CHICKWEED
(Stellaria media)

Also known as Starweed, Stitchwort, Adder's Mouth.

Description: This herb grows in hedges and ditches, in waste places, by the roadside, and in gardens. The stems are jointed with a line of fine hairs down one side only. The leaves grow opposite, are oval about $\frac{1}{2}$ inch long and $\frac{1}{4}$ inch broad, the lower ones on stalks, the upper springing from the stem; they spread upwards and escape being overshadowed by other broad-leaved plants. The flowers grow singly in the axils of the upper leaves, the petals are white with a silvery-grey tint and they look like stars.

Part used: The herb.

It is interesting that both wild and caged birds eat the seeds of this herb as well as the young tops and leaves. Pigs and rabbits like Chickweed; cows

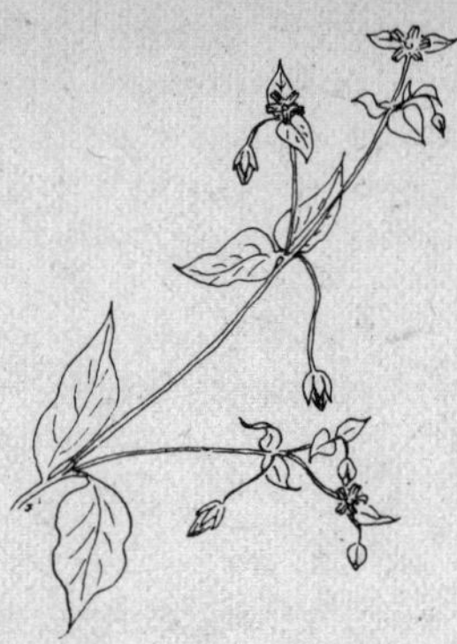

Chickweed

and horses will eat it; sheep are indifferent to it but goats refuse to touch it.

Fernie says: 'Fresh chickweed juice, as proved medicinally in 1893, produces sharp rheumatic pains and stitches in the head and eyes, with a general feeling of being bruised; also pressure about the liver and soreness there, with sensations of burning and of bilious indigestion. Subsequently the herb, when given in quite small doses of tincture or fresh juice, or infusion, has been found by its affinity to remove the train of symptoms just described, and to act most reliably in curing obstinate rheumatism.'

It should be thought of when pains are sharp and darting in any part of the body. It helps rheumatoid arthritis in different parts of the body; stiffness of joints; pains in shoulders and arms and in calves of legs. It also aids digestion. (Indigestion can be one of the contributing factors in the development of rheumatism.)

Directions for use: 1½ oz of the dried herb or 2 oz of the fresh herb should be boiled in 1½ pints of water down to 1 pint and when it is strained take half a teacupful every two or three hours.

A tea may be made by steeping a heaped teaspoonful of the dried herb for half an hour in a cup of boiling water. A cupful should be sipped slowly three or four times daily plus one at bedtime.

13.

COMFREY
(Symphytum officinale)

Also known as Blackwort, Nipbone, Knitbone, Consolida, Boneset.

Description: This herb grows by rivers and in moist places all over the country and in many gardens.

The plant has large hairy leaves (which are prickly), large at the base, getting smaller the higher they grow on the stalk, which is hollow and hairy. It grows about three feet with spikes of white flowers at the top. The root is brownish-black, deeply wrinkled.

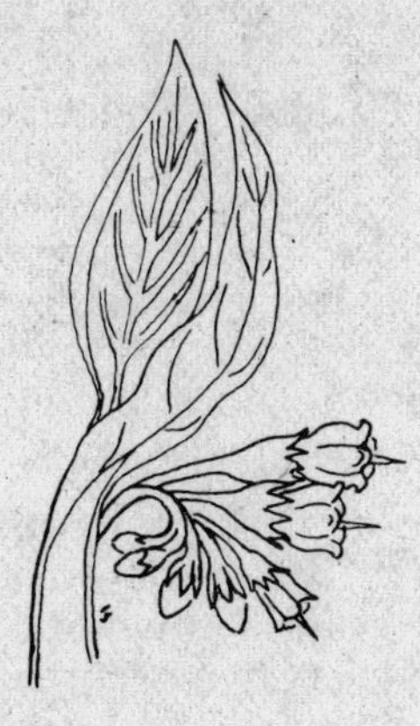

Comfrey

Part used: The root and leaves.

Formerly country people cultivated Comfrey because it was known to heal wounds and the many local names of the plant testify to its long reputation as a vulnerary herb; in the Middle Ages it was a famous remedy for broken bones.

The name Comfrey is a corruption of *con firma*, because of the uniting of bones it was thought to effect, and the botanical name Symphytum is derived from the Greek *symphyo*, 'to unite'.

Culpeper says: 'The roots of Comfrey taken fresh, beaten small and spread upon leather and laid upon any place troubled with the gout presently gives ease; and applied in the same manner eases pained joints. . . .'

Fernie says the whole plant, if beaten to a cataplasm, and applied hot as a poultice, has always been thought excellent for soothing pain in any tender, inflamed or suppurating part.

This herb greatly benefits arthritic conditions and circulation of the blood. It not only aids bones to knit together but soothes aching ones. It also acts on the joints generally.

Directions for use: One pint of boiling water should be poured on to 1 oz of the leaves and when it is cold and strained take a wineglassful three times daily.

14.

COUCH GRASS
(Agropyrum repens)

Also known as Twitchgrass, Triticum repens, Dog Grass or Quilch.

Description: It grows freely – far too freely – in gardens, where it is difficult to dislodge. The rhizome (or root) is tubular, about 1/10th inch in diameter, stiff, pale yellow, with nodes at intervals of about an inch.

Part used: The rhizome.

The synonym Dog-grass comes from its efficacy in curing dogs when they are ill. They are often to be seen searching for the rough leaves of Couchgrass which, when chewed, causes them to vomit and relieve their troubles.

Leon Petulengro states that this herb is very rich in Potassium, a most important mineral.

Couchgrass helps to obtain a better elimination of waste materials from the body through the kidneys and bladder and probably this is why it

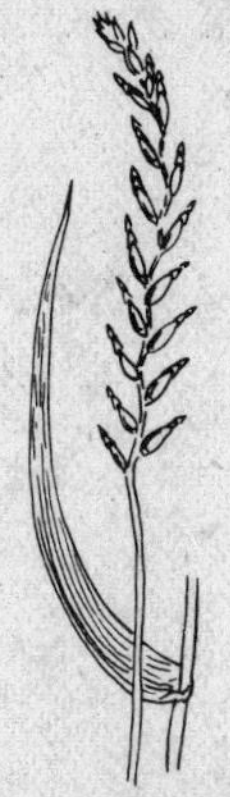

Couchgrass

can ease some of the pains of gout and rheumatism.

Directions for use: One quart of water should be poured on to the sliced dried root and boiled down to 1 pint. A wineglassful should then be taken three times daily.

15.

DAISY
(Bellis Perennis)

Also known as Bainwort, Lesser Consound and Bruisewort.

Description: The common daisy flowers from the earliest days of spring until late autumn and is well known on the lawns of many gardens! The flat leaves of this little plant grow so closely to the ground that nothing can grow underneath them.

Part used: The root and leaves.

There is a proverb which says: 'When you can put your foot on seven daisies, summer has come.'

During mediaeval times the Daisy was worn by

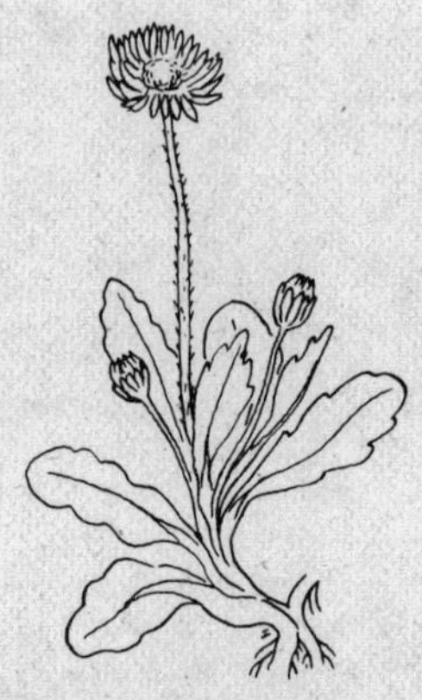

Daisy

18.

HORSERADISH
(Cochlearia Armoracia)

Description: It grows in ditches and odd corners where it increases by means of its roots, for it rarely produces seeds in this country. It is cultivated in many gardens, and is familiar as a condiment to accompany 'The Roast Beef of Old England'.

The root is white and cylindrical, about 1 foot long and ¾ inches in diameter. It can often be purchased fresh. Taste pungent, mustard-like; odour, when the root is scraped, recalling that of mustard, irritating to the nostrils and eyes.

Part used: The root.

This is said to be one of the five bitter herbs ordered to be eaten by the Jewish people during the Feast of the Passover, the other four being Coriander, Horehound, Lettuce and Nettle.

It contains quite a large proportion of sulphur and so is very useful in relieving chronic rheumatism.

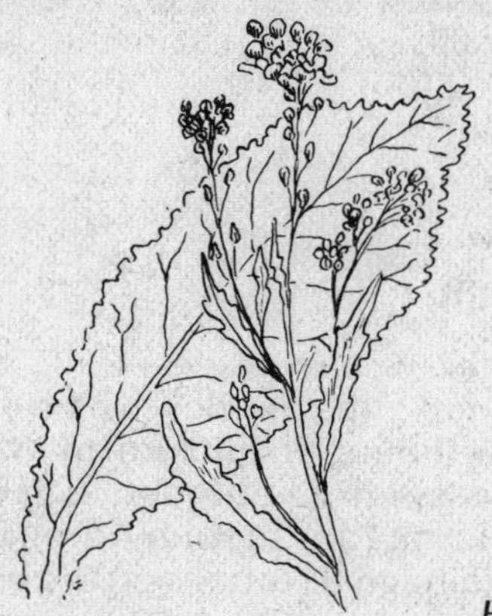

Horseradish

Gerard says of the root: 'If bruised and laid to the part grieved with the sciatica, gout, joynt-ache, or the hard swellings of the spleen and liver, it doth wonderfully help them all.'

When sliced across, the root of Horseradish will exude a few drops of a sweet juice which may be rubbed with advantage on parts of the body affected by rheumatism.

Directions for use:A compound made from the sliced fresh root, orange peel, a little nutmeg and Spirits of Wine helps chronic rheumatism. Leave standing overnight, then from one to two teaspoonsful may be taken in half a wineglassful of water after meals.

19.

JUNIPER
(Juniperis communis)

Description: This is a small shrub, the branches are thick with narrow, stiff leaves, of a bluish-green colour, sharp and prickly at the ends. The flowers are small and the berries round, green for the first year, and then purple or black, containing three-cornered seeds.

Part used: The berries.

Sprays of Juniper were frequently strewn on floors, so as to give out their pleasant odour when trodden down. The bedchamber of Queen Elizabeth I was sweetened with their scent.

The berries yield a large amount of sugar on boiling, and Linnaeus mentions that a decoction of these fruits, when fermented, forms a common beverage among the Swedes, who still eat Juniper berries at their meals in the form of a conserve.

Culpeper says of the berries: 'They strengthen the brain, fortify the sight, by strengthening the nerves they are good for agues, help the gout and

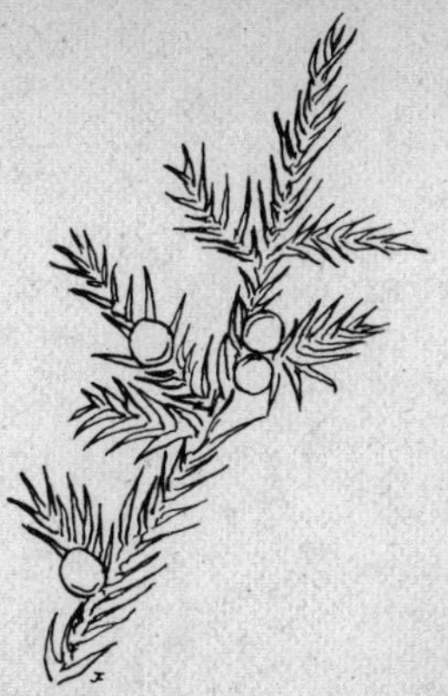

Juniper

sciatica and strengthen the limbs of the body.'

Juniper berries have disinfectant properties. They stimulate all functions of the body and increase the excretion of uric acid in the urine. Therefore they are recommended for all cases of arthritis and rheumatism.

Directions for use: An infusion is made by pouring 1 pint of boiling water on to 1 oz of the berries. When it is cold and strained take a wineglassful three times daily.

20.
LADY'S SLIPPER
(Cypripedium pubescens)

Also known as Lady's Shoe, Nerve-root, Noah's Ark, Yellow Lady's Slipper.

Description: This is one of the rarest and most beautiful of the British wild flowers; it is now almost extinct except in Yorkshire and Durham. It has a creeping root from which a downy stalk rises to about 12 inches. The leaves are broad, pale green and heavily ribbed and there are three or four on each stem. At the top of the stem there is

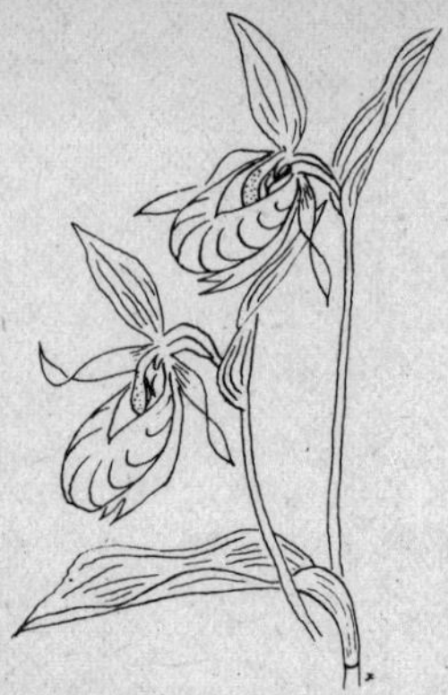

Lady's Slipper

one flower with reddish, sometimes twisted sepals, and a large inflated yellow lip, which attracts the bees. The flowers are large and showy and when newly open they have a very soft sweet perfume.

Part used: The root.

This remedy is an almost pure relaxant and helps the whole of the nervous system. It also allays pain.

Lady's Slipper should be thought of in all rheumatism of the neuralgic type and will help any sufferers from arthritis or rheumatism who are nervously upset, and suffer from tensions, which is not unusual.

Directions for use: One teaspoonful of the powdered root may be taken in sweetened water as a dose.

$\frac{1}{2}$-1 teaspoonful of the liquid extract may be taken in water three times daily.

knights at a tournament as an emblem of fidelity.

Gerard says: 'Daisies do mitigate all kinds of pain, especially in the joints, and gout proceeding from a hot humour. . . .'

This is an excellent remedy when there is muscular soreness, and the joints feel sore. Therefore if rheumatism or arthritic pains can be translated into 'soreness' the common Daisy should be given a trial.

Directions for use: One pint of boiling water should be poured on to 1 oz of the leaves or powdered root and when it is cool and strained take a wineglassful three times daily.

16.

DANDELION

(Taraxacum officinalis)

Also known as Blowball, Timetable, Wiggers, Swinesnout.

Description: This herb grows everywhere in pastures, meadows, on waste ground, and is well known as a weed in our gardens. The stems grow to a height of about 6 inches and there is one flower to each stem. The leaves have jagged edges which resemble the jaw of a lion fully supplied with teeth! The root is long, dark brown and very bitter, but not disagreeably so.

Part used: The leaves and root.

The flower of the dandelion when fully blown is named Priest's Crown (*Caput Monachi*), from the resemblance of its naked receptacle after the winged seeds have been blown away, to the smooth shorn head of a Roman cleric.

It was in the thirteenth century that the Dandelion was first mentioned by the Welsh. It

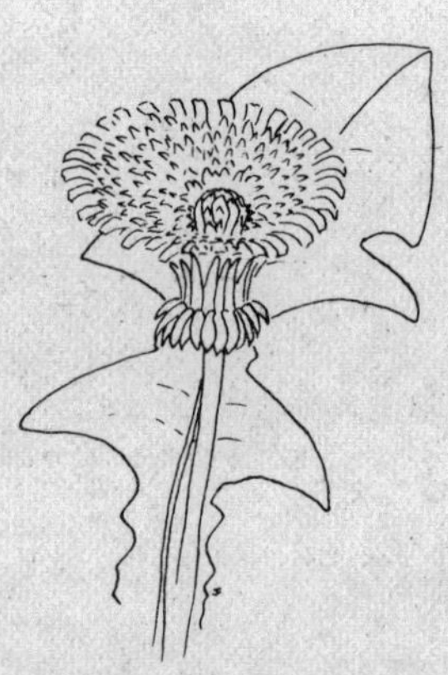

Dandelion

was greatly valued in the times of Gerard and Parkinson and is used extensively today.

Dandelion wine is very easily made and is good to drink, having a pleasant flavour.

This herb is good for a wide variety of illnesses and Culpeper says: 'You see here what virtues this common herb has, and that is the reason the French and Dutch so often eat them in the Spring; and if you now look a little further, you may see plainly without a pair of spectacles that foreign physicians are not so selfish as ours are, but more communicative of the virtues of plants to people.'

This herb has a tonic and diuretic effect and is slightly laxative. It contains iron, calcium, magnesium, potassium, silicon, sodium and mineral salts. It is a general stimulant to the system and will benefit all cases of rheumatism and arthritis.

Directions for use: 2 oz of the root or herb should be boiled in 1 quart of water down to 1 pint and when it is cool and strained take a wineglassful every three hours.

17.
GARLIC
(Allium Sativa)

Also known as Poor Man's Treacle, Churl's Treacle and by the Greeks, *Skorodon*.

Description: This herb is found in many gardens and it looks rather like an onion. The bulb consists of several combined cloves and has an odour much stronger than onions.

Part used: The bulb.

Garlic is still considered a delicacy in Egypt, where thousands of years ago the labourers taught the children of Israel to eat it.

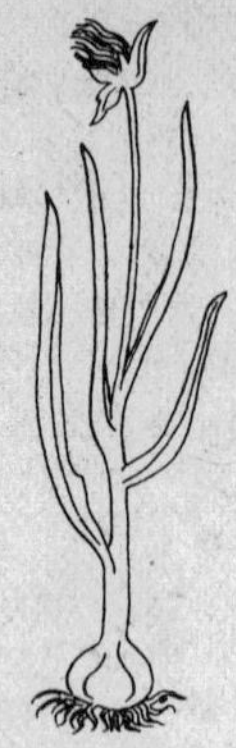

Garlic

This herb is mentioned in some of the old English lists of plants from the tenth to the fifteenth centuries and is described by herbalists of the sixteenth century onwards.

It is stated that it was grown in England before 1540.

The name is of Anglo-Saxon origin, being derived from gar – a spear, and lac – a plant, owing to the shape of the leaves.

A Mohammedan legend says that 'When satan stepped out from the Garden of Eden after the fall of man, Garlick sprang up from the spot where he placed his left foot and Onion from that where his right foot touched.'

Dr Fernie says: 'The pain of rheumatic parts may be made better by rubbing cut garlic on them.'

This herb helps to purify the blood and therefore must help all sufferers from arthritis and rheumatism.

Directions for use: A clove or two of garlic pounded with honey and taken two or three nights in succession is very good for rheumatism.

Capsules of garlic should be purchased and taken according to directions on the bottle.

21.

MEADOWSWEET
(Spirea ulmaria)

Also known as Queen of the Meadow, Bridewort, Lady of the Meadow.

Description: This is a common wild plant of the British Isles growing in meadows and woods. The root is red, thick and flabby. The stem is round and angular, erect, firm, pale green, but sometimes purple. The leaves are each composed of about three pairs of small leaves, which are set on each side of the mid-rib with the terminal one at the end. They are deep green on the upper side and whitish underneath. The flowers are small and white, standing so close together that the whole cluster seems to form one large flower. They have a very fragrant perfume.

Part used: The herb.

Meadowsweet, water mint and vervain were held most sacred by the Druids.

Gerard says: 'The leaves and the floures farre

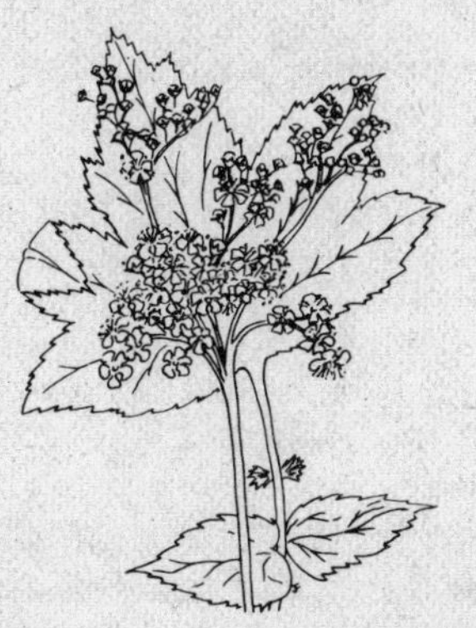

Meadowsweet

excell all other strewing herbes, for to decke up houses, to strew in chambers, halls and banqueting houses in the summer time; for the smell thereof makes the heart merrie, delighteth the senses; neither doth it cause headache, or lothsomenesse to meat, as some other sweet smelling herbes do.'

Meadowsweet is rich in iron and magnesium.

This is a good tonic in all cases of rheumatism. It promotes the appetite, strengthens the nerves and muscles and gives a sense of general well-being.

Directions for use: One pint of boiling water should be poured on to 1 oz of the dried herb. When it is cold and strained take a wineglassful three times daily.

22.

NETTLE
(Urtica dioica)

Also known as Stinging Nettle, Common Nettle.

Description: This herb grows on all waste ground. The stems are 2-3 feet high with opposite, stalked, oval leaves, serrated at the margins. The flowers are small, and green. It is recognized by its yellow,creeping root.

Part used: The flowers, leaves and seeds.

The word Nettle is derived from *net*, meaning something spun or sewn. Fibres of the Nettle are very similar to those of Hemp or Flax, and it was used for the same purposes, for making cloth of the finest texture down to the coarsest, such as sail-cloth, sacking, cordage, etc. In Hans Anderson's fairy tale of the Princess and the Eleven Swans, the coats she wove for them were made of Nettles.

When Germany and Russia ran short of cotton during World War I, the value of the Nettle as a substitute was at once recognized, and the greater and the smaller Nettle were especially selected for textiles.

Nettle tops should be gathered when young, cooked and eaten like spinach – they are delicious.

In Italy, where herb soups are popular, 'herb knodel' (or round balls made like dumplings in size and consistency) of Nettles are said to be nourishing and medicinal.

Nettles purify the blood, are alkaline and a solvent of uric acid; and therefore they are excellent for arthritic and rheumatic conditions. They are rich in iron, sulphur, potassium and sodium.

Directions for use: Nettle tea should be made by adding 1 oz of the herb or seed to 1 pint of boiling water. After at least five minutes it may be taken as tea or a wineglassful drunk three times daily.

5 drops of the tincture in a little water may be taken three times daily.

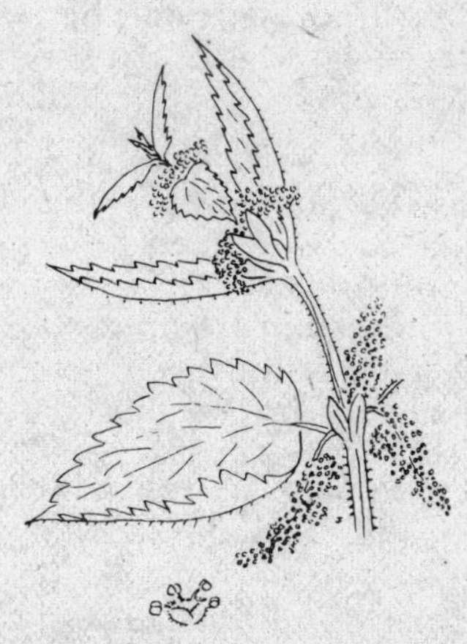

Nettle

23.
POTATO
(Solanum tuberosum)

Description: There is no need to describe this 'herb', which is known to everybody and grown by many.

Part used: The tubers.

The potato was introduced into England in 1586. Dr Fernie states that for a considerable time after this the potato tubers were grown only by men of fortune, as a delicacy; and the general cultivation of this vegetable was strongly opposed by the public, chiefly the Puritans, because no mention of it could be found in the Bible.

And again from Dr Fernie: 'The carriage of a small raw Potato in the trousers' pocket has been found preventive of rheumatism in a person predisposed thereto, probably by reason of the sulphur and the narcotic principles contained in the peel. Ladies in former times had their dresses supplied with special bags or pockets, in which to

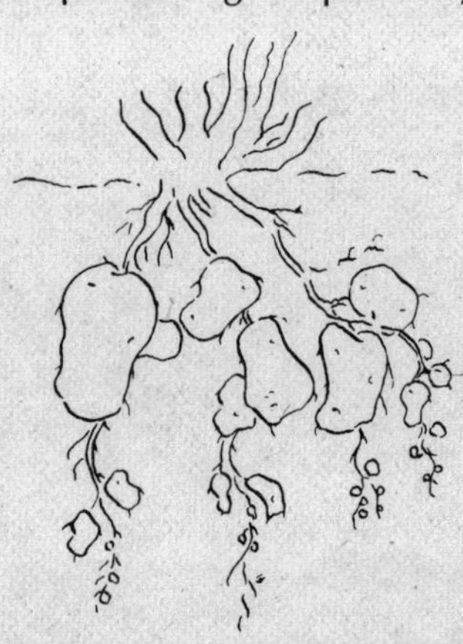

Potato

carry one or more small raw Potatoes about their person for avoiding rheumatism.'

The Potato contains citric acid, potash, and phosphoric acid just underneath the paper-thin skin; this is why potatoes should not be peeled, as these salts are then lost when they are eaten.

Potatoes are good for rheumatism of the joints, inflamed muscles and inflammation of the periosteum (the membrane covering) of the bones.

Directions for use: A wineglassful of potato juice should be taken first thing in the morning before anything is eaten.

A poultice from potatoes boiled in their skins, mixed with a little raw milk and applied to the painful part, is helpful. If heat cannot be tolerated allow potatoes to cool first.

24.

PRICKLY ASH
(Zanthoxylum Americanum)

Also known as Toothache Tree, Yellow Wood, Suterberry.

Description: This tree grows in America and Canada.

The Northern bark is in curved or quilled fragments, externally brownish-grey, with whitish patches, faintly furrowed. When broken it shows green in the outer and yellow in the inner part. Taste bitterish and very pungent, causing salivation. The Southern bark, which is usually sold, is 1/12th inch thick and has conical, corky spines sometimes 4/5th inches in height.

Part used: The bark and berries.

Dr F.H. England says: 'It has the power of getting right out to the small capillaries; that is why it is so good in cases of congestion, carrying blood

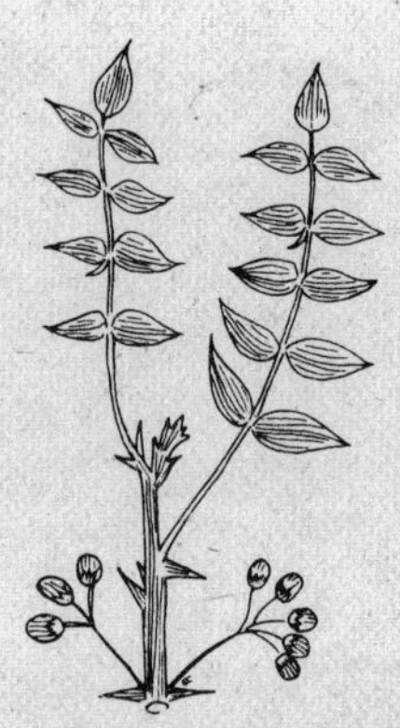

Prickly Ash

through the congested parts. It is a splendid remedy and not valued as it deserves to be. It is good in rheumatism because of its stimulating effect on the capillaries.'

This herb should be thought of when a general stimulant is required, especially in neuralgia and rheumatic complaints.

Directions for use: Liquid extract of the bark, ½-1 teaspoonful three times daily. Liquid extract of the berries, 10-30 drops in water three times daily.

An excellent prescription is as follows:

½ oz Prickly Ash bark
½ oz Guaiacum raspings
½ oz Buckbean herb
6 Cayenne pods

This should be boiled in 1½ pints of water down to 1 pint. When it is cool and strained take a wineglassful three or four times daily.

25.

RUE

(Ruta graveolens)

Also known as Garden Rue, Herb of Grace, Herbygrass, Ave-grass.

Description: This plant grows into a sturdy little shrub that is very hardy, on poor soil in many English gardens. It is bushy with small leaves of soft, bluish-green, and has small yellow flowers at the top of the stems. It is one of the 'bitter' herbs and has a very aromatic scent.

Part used: The herb.

Rue is first mentioned by Turner in 1562 and has become one of the best known, and widely used Simples in Herbal Medicine.

The name *Ruta* is from the greek *reuo* 'to set free' because it has such a variety of uses.

It was highly thought of by the Ancients; Hippocrates commended it; the Greeks wrote about it and in the Middle Ages it was considered (in many parts of Europe) as a powerful defence

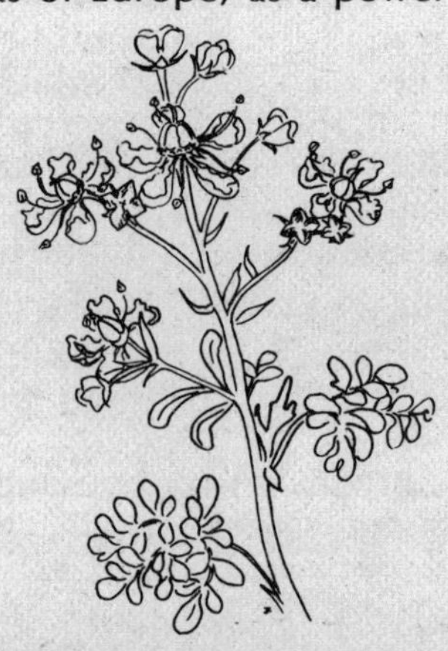

Rue

against witches! It was also thought to bestow second sight.

Culpeper recommends it for sciatica and pains in the joints, if the latter be anointed with it.

Infusions of this herb help to remove formation of deposits in tendons and joints and therefore it is very useful in the treatment of arthritis.

Directions for use: A small wineglassful of the infusion, made by pouring 1 pint of boiling water on to 1 oz of the herb and allowing it to stand for a few minutes, should be taken three times daily.

26.

WHITE BRYONY
(Bryonia dioica)

Also known as: English Mandrake, Bryonia, Mandragora, Wild Vine, Lady's Seal.

Description: This plant is a native of Europe and often found in England, but rarely in Scotland.

It is a climbing plant with curling tendrils. The leaves are large, growing alternately up the stem, shaped like the palm of the hand, with five toothed lobes. They are rough on both sides and supported by long stalks. The flowers are in small clusters growing from the axils of the leaves. The plant produces a green berry which turns orange and finally red. The stems are from 5-6 feet high, branched and covered with small hairs. The root is 1-2 feet long or more, branched, 1-3 inches in diameter. It is white externally and internally.

Part used: The root.

The White Bryony is botanically a cucumber growing freely by our roadsides and often called The White Vine.

The name Bryony is two thousand years old and comes from the Greek *bruein*, 'to shoot forth rapidly'.

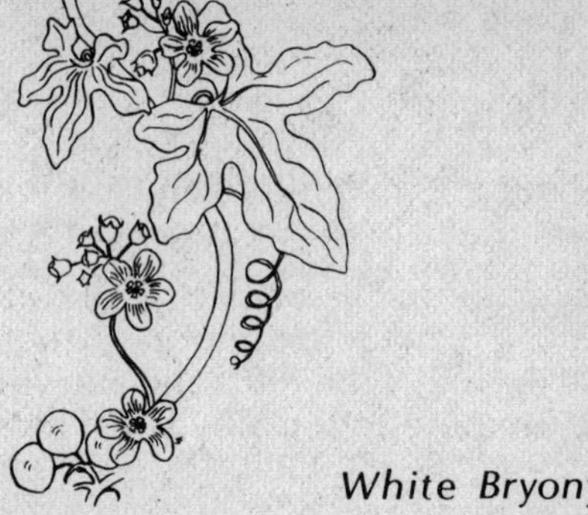

White Bryony

It was well known in the fourteenth century as Wild Nep and used as an antidote to leprosy. The juice from the fleshy root was used by the Greeks and Romans, prescribed by Galen and Dioscorides, and later by Gerard as a purgative.

Bryony has been praised for helping sciatica, rheumatism and lumbago, and should be thought of when the joints are red, swollen and hot, and when any aches and pains are worse for movement.

Directions for use: $\frac{1}{4}$-$\frac{1}{2}$ teaspoonful of the liquid extract in water should be taken three times daily for two or three weeks.

27.

YELLOW DOCK
(Rumex Crispus)

Also known as Sour Dock, Curled Dock, Garden Patience.

Description: This herb grows freely in roadside ditches and on waste ground. The leaves are narrow and oblong, and crisped at the margins. Sepals hang down from short individual stalks from the main stem in groups of five or six. The root occurs in short shrivelled pieces $\frac{3}{4}$-1 inch long, brown, rough and wrinkled.

Part used: The root.

The generic name of several Docks is *rumex* from the Hebrew *rumach*, a 'spear'.

Dr Vassar, an old American herbalist, says that the Yellow Dock is an iron carrier.

It is a very good tonic and tones up the entire system. Also it is a blood purifier and laxative and therefore all patients suffering from arthritis or

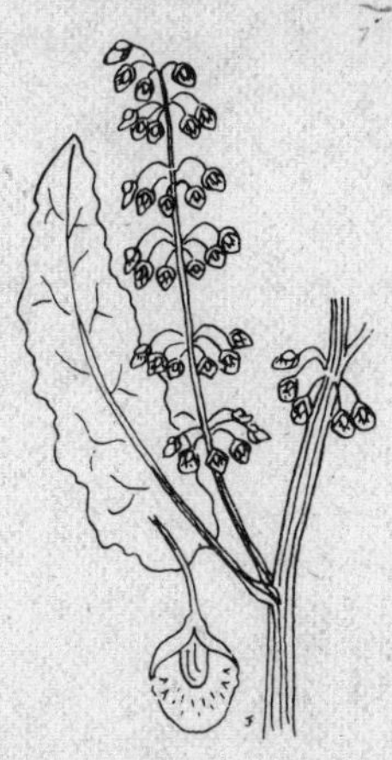

Yellow Dock

rheumatism will benefit from a course of this herbal medicine.

Directions for use: One pint of boiling water should be added to 1 oz of the powdered root; when it is cold and strained a wineglassful may be taken three times daily.

28.
SUPPLEMENTARY ADVICE

Diet

The intake of correct food plays a very important role in the treatment of rheumatic diseases.

It is because the body produces excess acids that many of these aches and pains come to the fore, and so, apart from the purifying herbs, we must examine the daily diet.

One of the most common errors today is the over-indulgence in sugar. Sweets, cakes, buns, candies and biscuits are easy 'fillers', but they are all harmful. The refining of sugar to obtain the white varieties, removes at least a great proportion of mineral salts and nutritive elements from the crude substance. When taken into the body refined sugar causes an acid reaction, and it leeches the system of calcium and robs it of quantities of the B vitamins which are necessary for good health.

A little honey may be taken or added to any foods which really require sweetening, but it should not be forgotten that the body can convert about 60 per cent. of the proteins eaten into glucose, which is blood sugar, as is necessary. People in far away places (for example, the Eskimos, who rarely, if ever, eat sweet things because they are unobtainable, never suffer from low blood sugar because they eat plenty of protein.

It should be remembered that fruits contain natural sugar.

Salt tends to encourage the pains of arthritis. It should be avoided except for a very little sea-salt in cooking, if desired. Many natural foods contain minute amounts of salt, which are acceptable to the body and in most instances this is all that is necessary.

Wholemeal bread only should be consumed and never bread made from white flour. The roughage in the 100 per cent. wholemeal helps the bowels to function efficiently.

People over middle-age very often do not need to eat bread at all. Too much starch is often included in the normal diet and this should be reduced by avoiding all white flour products.

Starches and sugars help to make up carbohydrates, which give the body heat and energy. But excessive carbohydrates produce acidity and so starches, as well as sugars, should be cut to the minimum. However, some starches in their natural form are nourishing and more easily digested, such as wholemeal bread, 'jacket potatoes, brown rice and really ripe bananas, but the intake should be limited. All cakes, puddings, buns, white bread, custard powder, macaroni and pasta should be rejected.

The following list of alkaline foods should be helpful in the preparation of healthy meals.

Almonds
Apples
Apricots
Beetroot
Buttermilk
Black molasses
Cabbage
Carrots
Cauliflower
Celery
Cherries
Citrus fruits
Cream cheese
Cucumber
Currants
Dates
Grapes
Lettuce
Mushrooms
Non-pasteurized milk
Olives
Onions
Parsnips
Peaches
Pears
Pineapple
Potatoes
Radishes
Raisins
Raspberries
Skimmed milk
Strawberries
Turnips

Foods should never be cooked in aluminium pots. Instead, stainless steel, enamel and toughened china or glass ovenware should be used. Food should be grilled, steamed or baked, it should not be fried.

A salad should be taken every day, consisting of a combination of some of the following: lettuce, grated raw beetroot, grated raw carrot, shredded raw cabbage, celery, cucumber, mushrooms, olives, radishes, tomatoes, watercress, mustard and cress.

A little fresh dressing may be added, made from a tablespoonful of lemon juice and three of sunflower seed oil, mixed in a bottle with a saltspoonful of mustard, a saltspoonful of brown sugar and a little freshly milled black pepper. This makes a very appetizing lunch or evening meal with a little cream cheese or some nuts or an egg as protein. Some fresh fruit should follow.

For the second meal of the day, according to when the salad is taken, there may be a choice of lamb, chicken or white fish, with one or two green vegetables, some steamed carrots or parsnips, and a jacket potato. If vegetarian, then one of the savouries given in the variety of vegetarian cook books should supply the protein. This may be followed by apple snow, baked apples, yogurt, pears (raw or stewed), or stewed fresh or dried apricots, etc.

Fruit juices may be taken mid-morning and/or mid-afternoon. Cucumber, carrot and apple are very beneficial. Cucumber juice can be expressed and there are one or two excellent apple juices already bottled on the market which are pure and delicious. For those possessing a juice extractor a combination of these three juices is excellent and a wineglassful once or twice daily would be very beneficial.

Watercress is especially good as it contains iodine, iron, potash, sulphur and phosphate salts.

There are some good recipes for watercress soup, which could be taken before the cooked meal.

Alternatively a little vegetable soup may be taken before the cooked meal, or during mid-morning in cold weather.

Potassium broth is an excellent mid-morning or pre-evening meal drink in winter-time, as potassium is very important for sufferers from rheumatism.

The following is a good recipe:

Carrot or Turnip
Spinach or Watercress
Onion or Leeks
Tomato, fresh or bottled
Celery or tablespoonful Celery Seed crushed
Parsley, $\frac{1}{4}$ cup only

Place in a stainless steel or suitable saucepan with 5 pints of cold water, bring to the boil and simmer for at least 20 minutes.

Foods rich in potassium are:

Celery
Apples
Jacket potatoes
Peas
Watercress
Almonds
Cottage cheese
Lamb
Grapes
Lentils
Raisins
Figs
Whole wheat

A cup of herbal or weak China tea may be taken during the afternoon.

Good, health-giving meals can be made up from the details given in this section, and in most cases, great benefit is derived, in a comparatively short time.

Vitamins

There is no doubt that everybody needs a course of 'natural' vitamins in capsule or tablet form at intervals, due to the fact that the food obtained today is deficient in both vitamins and minerals necessary for good health.

It is not recommended, however, that vitamins should be taken for an indefinite period, neither should it be assumed that by taking various vitamins all forms of disease will vanish! Too many are almost as bad as too few.

Vitamin C. is the most important for patients suffering from the various forms of rheumatism. It has been found that sick people recover more quickly when they are taking vitamin C and tests show that toxins combine with this vitamin and together they are excreted in the urine.

The question is always asked, 'How much shall I take?' and this is very difficult to answer. The body cannot store Vitamin C and obviously from the foregoing, more is needed when a patient is sick than when healthy. It must be replenished daily and the best source is from our foods; if only we could be sure that they are grown organically and do, in fact, contain the elements they should! The foods richest in Vitamin C are:

Rose hips	Black currants
Pimentos	Grapefruit
Turnip tops	Broccoli leaf
Brussel sprouts	Parsley
Strawberries	Watercress
Oranges	Dandelion leaves
Cabbage	Kale
Sweet melon	

In addition to a diet rich in the foods containing vitamin C, two or three capsules daily for a month or six weeks will very often bring about an improvement.

It is wise to consider the multi vitamins – these are usually capsules containing all the vitamins – and a course of one of the 'natural' ones for a month or six weeks will give a boost to the body as a whole and is of particular value to the nervous system.

Epsom Salts Baths

These baths can be very helpful and soothing to patients, providing *they do not suffer from any heart condition or high blood-pressure.*

The patient should sit for ten minutes in a bath half filled with hot water to which has been added 1-2 lb of crude Epsom salts. The temperature should be controlled to suit each patient. A loofah or skin brush should be used throughout and the skin constantly brushed to remove waste products which are eliminated through the pores of the skin. If this is not done, debris clogs the pores and no more elimination can take place.

After ten minutes the water should be emptied away, making sure that the bath is cleaned of any deposits, and the body then washed all over in fresh, warm water. A pure soap may be used.

This bath should be taken just before getting into bed between flannelette sheets or thin blankets.

If a full bath is not acceptable, then compresses can be helpful. A piece of linen should be dipped into a bowl of cold water containing a handful of Epsom salts. When wrung out it should be applied to the affected part and immediately covered with a woollen scarf or piece of blanket and fastened in place. If this does not warm up the area at once by stimulating the circulation, the linen should be removed and the skin washed in warm water, otherwise a chill may follow. If the part being treated soon becomes warm, the compress should be left on all night.

Compresses should be applied twice a week, and if the condition is bad, they should be used in addition to baths, providing the latter can be tolerated. The linen should be thoroughly washed, boiled and dried between each compress.

Some patients are able to take foot-baths even though they cannot manage full water baths. 4 oz of Epsom salts should be added to a bowl of hot water and the feet immersed in it for about fifteen minutes, more hot water being added when necessary, to keep up the temperature. Again, the feet should be rubbed frequently with a brush or loofah, and then washed in fresh warm water, and a little vegetable oil rubbed into the skin.

The patient should go to bed or keep very warm after the foot bath as, usually, the body sweats from the heat generated from the feet.

Exercise

This is very important for all sufferers from arthritis and rheumatism, but it must be taken according to the severity of the aches and pains, as under no circumstances must it cause strain. Some patients, of course, cannot take any exercise at all, but, fortunately, these are in the minority.

Walking in the fresh air is excellent, but care must be taken not to go too far, because physical overtiredness can cause more pain. The patient should walk as far as he feels capable of doing, comfortably, at his own pace, and this may vary from day to day. Whilst in the fresh air he should breathe in deeply, so taking oxygen into the lungs.

If the trouble is in the hands and fingers, in addition to the daily walk, it is a good thing to clench and open the fists, and move the fingers, to stop them from getting too stiff. A good aid is to handle a soft ball and squeeze it as hard as possible. A set of exercises repeated two or three times daily regularly is very beneficial.

Lying flat on the bed and moving the legs as though pedalling a bicycle is helpful if the trouble is in the muscles of the legs. This should be done ten times, then a rest taken before 'pedalling' for another ten times, and so on. It should be done slowly and without strain.

If there are aches and pains in the neck and across the shoulders, place the hands on the shoulders with the elbows pointing to the floor.

Now keeping the shoulders as still as possible move the arms up, back and down so that the tips of the elbows rotate in circles – the hands are still on the shoulders. Repeat this slowly half a dozen times and then reverse the direction and take the arms back, up and forward. Repeat this six times.

Again it must be emphasized that exercises must not be tiring. They should be increased as the body accommodates, otherwise they could hinder rather than help the condition.

Never exercise any part of the body if the pain is made worse.

Relaxation

This is essential for *everybody* in these days of tensions and strains, but more especially for sick people, and those with arthritic or rheumatic troubles can derive great benefit from consciously relaxing.

When sitting in a chair it is wise, at intervals, to make oneself alert as to what is happening. It may be that the patient is sitting with clenched fists; he may have his shoulders and neck taut, or he may be sitting with his back like a ram-rod tensed up. When any fault of this nature is found it should be rectified, the part freed from strain and 'loosened'.

Chores in the kitchen often produce tensions in the housewife. Cutting up fruits or vegetables, stirring mixtures and beating will cause tension across the neck and shoulders, particularly if the working top is not at the right height. These jobs should be done for a shorter period, with rests in between. A good exercise to help this tension is given in the last section.

It is always good to relax in bed and conscious relaxation often promotes sleep. The patient should lie flat on the bed and first think about the head. It should be dropped heavily on to the pillow. Then the eyes, and mouth should be thought of in turn to make sure they are not tensed. The neck and shoulders are next on the list – they should be loosened and allowed to sink limply on to the bed. Every part of the body from the head to the toes should be thought of in this way – even the fingers and toes. Very often before the exercise is completed, the patient is fast asleep – in a relaxed state!

If the advice given in this book is followed, for a reasonable time, the general level of health will be raised, and in most cases a feeling of well-being will follow, even if cure is not possible.

THERAPEUTIC INDEX

Arthritis, Agrimony, Ash, Bladderwrack, Burdock, Celery, Dandelion, Garlic, Juniper, Meadowsweet, Nettle, Prickly Ash, Rue, Yellow Dock.
Arthritis, Rheumatoid, Chickweed.
Blood Purifier, Burdock, Centaury, Garlic, Nettle, Yellow Dock.
Bones, Aching, Comfrey.
Elimination, Through Bladder and Kidneys, Couchgrass, Dandelion.
Elimination of Uric Acid, Juniper.
Gout, Angelica, Couchgrass
Joints, Hot, White Bryony.
Joints, Painful, Ash.
Joints, Red, White Bryony.
Joints, Rheumatism of, Comfrey, Potato.
Joints, Sore, Daisy.
Joints, Stiff, Chickweed.
Joints, Swollen, White Bryony.
Laxative, Ash, Dandelion, Yellow Dock.
Limbs, Aching, Black Cohosh.
Lumbago, Buckbean, White Bryony.
Muscles of Back, Painful, Black Cohosh.
Muscles, Belly of Painful, Black Cohosh.
Muscles, Inflammation of, Potato
Muscles of Neck, Painful, Black Cohosh.
Muscular Soreness, Black Cohosh, Daisy.
Pains in Arms, Chickweed.
Pains in Calves, Chickweed.
Pains, Darting, Chickweed.
Pains, Sharp, Chickweed
Pains in Shoulders, Chickweed.
Pains Worse, Movement, White Bryony.
Rheumatism, Agrimony, Ash, Bladderwrack, Burdock, Celery, Couchgrass, Dandelion, Garlic,

Juniper, Meadowsweet, Nettle, Prickly Ash, White Bryony, Yellow Dock.

Rheumatism, Chronic, Angelica, Buckbean, Horseradish.

Rheumatism, Intercostal, Black Cohosh.

Rheumatism, Muscular, Burdock, Centaury.

Rheumatic Neuralgia, Horseradish, Lady's Slipper.

Sciatica, White Bryony.

Tonic, White Bryony.

Other recommended books . . .

ARTHRITIS:

HELP IN YOUR OWN HANDS

Helen B. MacFarlane. No one, however "crippled" by chronic arthritis, need wait impotently for the disease to complete its destructive work. Author progressed from semi-invalidism to mobility through practising techniques—explained in this book—which are designed to stop deterioration and activate the healing process! Her success could be applied to almost anyone suffering from osteoarthritis, fibrositis, or other rheumatic diseases. *Contents include:* Electric massagers; Exercises; Vitamin deficiencies; Cortisone-producing diet; Importance of moderation; Connection between arthritis and "negative personality"; The "rheumatoid factor"; Ionizers; Cultured milk; minerals; Cod liver oil therapy; Fats; Helpful organizations; Aids and appliances; Useful hints.

HERBAL TEAS FOR HEALTH AND HEALING

Ceres. *Illustrated.* Over a hundred tea-making herbs are described in this delightful book. Some are slightly stimulating, others are tonics for restoring the system to complete health. Many can 'lift' melancholy and depression; others are nocturnal and daytime tranquillizers, and there are teas to alleviate pain and clear the skin, also herbal infusions for external uses as poultices and skin-tonics. *Includes:* Carminative teas 'for comforting the stomacke'; Cosmetic teas 'for helping to beautify the skin'; Pain-killing teas 'for allaying the agony'; Febrifuge teas 'to allay the fever'; Teas to induce sleep 'and to help settle obstreporous spirits'.

A DOCTOR'S PROVEN NEW HOME CURE FOR ARTHRITIS

Giraud W. Campbell D.O. Reveals a radical 7-day programme for ending osteo *and* rheumatoid arthritis and regaining *normal* joint movement. This amazing drugless therapy utilizes ingredients which may already be in your kitchen! Dr Campbell has cured hundreds of arthritic sufferers by this method, *including those who were bedridden. Part contents:* How to clean your insides to begin the purification process; Sixteen poisons that contribute to your arthritis; Seven-day menu for a new pain-free life; Your most valuable foods; How to sidestep the pain of arthritis permanently.

THE ALLERGY CONNECTION

Barbara Paterson. Did you know that smoking and the Pill are both prime instigators of migraine? Or that milk, cheese, bread, sugar, chocolate, tea, coffee or even oranges could each be a root cause of many apparently unrelated illnesses? Read here how nineteen leading specialists track down the hidden causes of illness in hundreds of new patients every year enabling them to lead new lives, free of tranquillizers, sleeping tablets and powerful drugs. In this book Barbara Paterson traces the course of her investigations into allergy related problems. She gives accounts of remarkable case histories where sufferers have been permanently cured of illnesses traditional medicine had been unable to either diagnose or alleviate.

THE ALLERGY PROBLEM

WHY PEOPLE SUFFER AND WHAT SHOULD BE DONE

Vicky Rippere MA. Explores the difficulties of allergic people (based on a nation-wide survey), and offers guidance to victims and their families. As our physical environment and food supply become more contaminated with the residues of so-called technological progress, people who develop symptoms upon exposure to these residues will find it progressively harder to avoid them. *Includes:* Food allergy — a personal account; Allergens; Help-seeking; Limitations on everyday activities resulting from allergy; Social reactions to allergic people; Special worries of allergic people; Sufferers' views on social changes; Summary and conclusions; Food allergy survey.

E FOR ADDITIVES

The Complete E-Number Guide

Everyone who is concerned about the quality of food they eat, whether they have health problems or not, will want a copy of this invaluable book. In E For Additives **Maurice Hanssen** tells us everything there is to know about each of the E-Numbers listed on food packets — what they are, where they come from, and what the possible adverse effects are. The facts uncovered are both fascinating and helpful. We learn that

- E-Numbers that are preservatives are essential for cutting the risks of food poisoning.
- E-Numbers that are emulsifiers and stabilizers can be used to disguise the amount of fat in meat — thus there can be some 40 per cent of fat in a meat product which looks like solid lean.
- E-Numbers that are polyphosphates used to 'tenderize' cured meats are in reality a way of adding water (and therefore weight) to the food.

Here, for the first time, we are given full exact information — an essential and indispensable reference book for everyone concerned about what they are eating.

SELENIUM

THE ESSENTIAL TRACE ELEMENT YOU MIGHT NOT BE GETTING ENOUGH OF

Alan Lewis. Here are the facts about this essential mineral — one of the most vital of the twenty or so trace elements that the body needs — but, because Britain is a low-selenium area, most of us don't get enough of it. This book reveals the link between low-selenium levels and the incidence of ill-health. It includes exciting new material on the use of selenium in the treatment of rheumatism and arthritis, and shows how it is beneficial in the treatment of heart disease and cancer. Explores its remarkable potential and gives vital information on the role of selenium in a balanced and healthy diet.

THE VITAMIN C CONNECTION

GETTING WELL AND STAYING WELL WITH VITAMIN C

Drs Emanuel Cheraskin, W. Marshall Ringsdorf Jr & Emily L. Sisley. Vital information on how Vitamin C enhances immune mechanisms, fights cancer and heart disease, protects against flu and bronchitis. 25 years of research proves that Vitamin C does more than prevent the common cold! *Contents include:* How not to be bugged by infections; Vitamin C — the natural healer; Pain and Vitamin C; Sugar is sweet — except in diabetes; The two C's in cancer; Seeing with C; It's *not* all in your mind!; Addiction plus Vitamin C equals no addiction; A 'C' full of smiles.